The World of Steaks

A Collection of 100+ Irresistible Recipes That You Can Prepare at Home Even if You Are a Beginner Cook

David Bluford

SPECIAL DISCLAIMER

All the information's included in this book are given for instructive, informational and entertainment purposes, the author can claim to share very good quality recipes but is not headed for the perfect data and uses of the mentioned recipes, in fact the information's are not intent to provide dietary advice without a medical consultancy.

The author does not hold any responsibility for errors, omissions or contrary interpretation of the content in this book.

It is recommended to consult a medical practitioner before to approach any kind of diet, especially if you have a particular health situation, the author isn't headed for the responsibility of these situations and everything is under the responsibility of the reader, the author strongly recommend to preserve the health taking all precautions to ensure ingredients are fully cooked.

All the trademarks and brands used in this book are only mentioned to clarify the sources of the information's and to describe better a topic and all the trademarks and brands mentioned own their copyrights and they are not related in any way to this document and to the author.

This document is written to clarify all the information's of publishing purposes and cover any possible issue.

This document is under copyright and it is not possible to reproduce any part of this content in every kind of digital or printable document. All rights reserved.

© Copyright 2021 David Bluford. All rights reserved.

Table Of Contents

Barbecued Steak Strips	1
Pace ® Sirloin Steak Ole	2
Merlot-Peppercorn Steak Sauce	3
Grilled Salmon Steaks with Savory Blueberry Sauce	4
Rib Eye Steaks with a Soy and Ginger Marinade	5
Dad's Steak Rub	6
Chicken Fried Venison Steaks	7
Swordfish Steaks with Arugula and Basil Sauce	8
Venison Burger and Steak Chili	9
Korean Marinated Flank Steak	10
Mushroom Round Steak	11
Tangy Ham Steak	12
Beer and Brown Sugar Steak Marinade	13
Salisbury Steak Deluxe	14
Oven-Fried Ranch Steak	15
Cubed Steak and Wild Rice	16
Cube Steak Parmigiana	17
Sirloin Steak with Garlic Butter	18
Sweet Grilled Steak Bites	19
Braised Skirt Steak with Artichoke	20
Brandied Pepper Steak	21
Chicken Pepper Steak	22
Salisbury Steak	23
Steak Salad (Ranen Salad)	24
Easy Minute Steaks	25
Steak Burritos	26
Chicken Fried Steak III	27
Chinese Pepper Steak	28
Teriyaki Rib Eye Steaks	29
Steak 'N' Vegetable Soup	30
Peppered Steak with Blackberry Sauce	31
Wasabi Encrusted Tuna Steaks	32
Grilled Salmon Steaks Italian-Style	33
Paprika Chili Steak	34
Steak House Au Gratin Potatoes	35

Table Of Contents

Thyme-Rubbed Steaks with Sauteed Mushrooms	36
Spicy Lime-Cilantro Marinated Flank Steak	37
Peanut Sesame Rib-Eye Steak	38
Ostrich Steaks with Calvados Sauce	39
Willy's Juicy Steak	40
Flank Steak Pinwheels	41
Japanese Sesame Steak Sauce	42
Luau Beef Tenderloin Steaks	43
Bangin' Steak Rub	44
Creamy Sliced Steak and Potatoes	45
Flat Iron Steak with Mushrooms	46
Salsa Steak For One	47
Pork Steaks	48
Steak and Rice	49
Flat Iron Steak and Spinach Salad	50
Teriyaki Steak	51
Berdean's Cube Steak	52
Finger Steaks	53
Stir-Fried Steak and Veggies	54
Pineapple-Green Onion Salsa with Cook's Ham Steak	55
Philly Steak Salad	56
Beef Pepper Steak	57
Flash-In-The-Pan Pepper Steak	58
Marinated Venison Steaks	59
Southwest Steak Bites	60
Saskatchewan City Steak Soup	61
Grilled Rib Eye Steaks	62
Bloody Mary Steaks with Green Olive Butter	63
Lavender Pork Steaks	64
Red Wine Reduction Steak Sauce	65
Spinach Steak Pinwheels	66
Marinated Flank Steak	67
Perfect Flat Iron Steak	68
Steak 'N' Onion Pie	69
Cumin Lamb Steaks with Smashed Potatoes, Wilted Spinach and	70

Table Of Contents

Rock's T-Bone Steaks	71
Firecracker Flank Steak	72
Special Salmon Steaks	73
Baked Fake Steak with Gravy	74
Marinade for Steak I	75
Sicilian Style Steak	76
Chicken Fried Steak II	77
Coffee Marinated Steak	78
Smoky Steak Marinade	79
Rosemary Steak	80
Seasoned Flank Steak	81
Doreen's Steak Marinade	82
Spinach-Stuffed Steak	83
Mock Chicken Fried Steak	84
Marinated Sirloin Steak	85
Creole Pan-Fried Flat Iron Steak	86
Lemon Basil Pesto Flat Iron Steak	87
Fiesta Grilled Ham Steak	88
Pepper Steak and Rice	89
Tasty Tuna Steak	90
John's Mango Steak	91
Sesame Sirloin Steak	92
President Ford's Braised Eye Round Steak	93
Slow-Cooked Flank Steak	94
Kicky Steak Strips with Rice	95
Steak Salad	96
Halibut Steaks	97
Steaks With Roquefort Sauce	98
Steakhouse Wheat Bread for the Bread Machine	99
Cheddar Mushroom Pork Steaks	100
Steak on a Stick	101
Comforting Cube Steaks	102

Barbecued Steak Strips

Ingredients

1 pound boneless beef sirloin steak, cut 1/2 inch strips
1 tablespoon vegetable oil
1 cup barbecue sauce
2 tablespoons honey
1 teaspoon sugar

Directions

In a large skillet, brown steak in oil over medium-high heat; drain. Combine the barbecue sauce, honey and sugar; pour over meat. Bring to a boil. Reduce heat; simmer, uncovered, for 10-15 minutes or until the sauce is slightly thickened and meat is tender.

PaceB® Sirloin Steak Ole

Ingredients

1 1/2 pounds boneless beef sirloin steak or beef top round steak
1 (16 ounce) jar PaceB® Picante Sauce or Chunky Salsa

Directions

Lightly oil the grill rack and heat the grill to medium. Grill the steak for 20 minutes for medium-rare or to desired doneness, turning the steak over halfway through cooking and brushing often with 1 cup picante sauce.

Let stand for 10 minutes before slicing. Serve with additional picante sauce.

Merlot-Peppercorn Steak Sauce

Ingredients

1 tablespoon butter
4 mushrooms, sliced
1 clove garlic, minced
2 tablespoons whole black peppercorns
1/4 cup Merlot wine
1 tablespoon balsamic vinegar
3 tablespoons Worcestershire sauce
1/2 teaspoon minced fresh rosemary

Directions

Melt butter in a saucepan over medium heat. Stir in the mushrooms, garlic, and peppercorns, and saute until the mushrooms are tender. Pour in the wine, balsamic, and Worcestershire sauce, increase the heat to medium-high, and reduce by 1/3. Stir in the rosemary and cook for 1 to 2 minutes until fragrant.

Grilled Salmon Steaks with Savory Blueberry

Ingredients

1/2 cup chicken stock
1/4 cup balsamic vinegar
1/4 cup orange juice
1 teaspoon honey
1 tablespoon cornstarch
1/4 cup chicken stock
1 cup fresh blueberries
2 teaspoons chopped fresh chives
4 (6 ounce) salmon steaks
2 tablespoons olive oil
salt and pepper to taste

Directions

Pour 1/2 cup chicken stock, vinegar, orange juice, and honey into a saucepan. Bring to a boil over high heat, then reduce heat to medium. Dissolve cornstarch in 1/4 cup of chicken stock, and stir into the simmering sauce. Cook and stir until the sauce thickens and turns clear, 1 to 2 minutes. Stir in the blueberries and chives, and keep warm over low heat.

Preheat grill to medium high-heat.

Brush salmon with oil, and season to taste with salt and pepper. Grill until the fish flakes easily with a fork, about 3 to 4 minutes per side. Serve with blueberry sauce.

Rib Eye Steaks with a Soy and Ginger Marinade

Ingredients

1/2 cup soy sauce
1/4 cup real maple syrup
6 cloves garlic, minced
1 tablespoon grated fresh ginger
1 teaspoon mustard powder
1/2 teaspoon sesame oil
1/4 teaspoon hot pepper sauce
1/2 cup beer
4 (10 ounce) beef rib eye steaks

Directions

In a medium size mixing bowl, combine soy sauce, maple syrup, garlic, ginger root, mustard powder, sesame oil, and Tabasco sauce; mix well to blend. Now add beer, and stir lightly to mix.

Prepare steaks by scoring any fatty outside areas on steak with a knife, (this prevents the steaks from curling when barbecuing). Place steaks in a casserole dish, and pour marinade over. Using a fork, punch holes in steaks so that the marinade penetrates into the steaks. Turn steaks over, and repeat punching holes.

Cover with clear wrap or foil, and let marinate in the refrigerator for at least 1 hour or longer. You can also refrigerate and marinate overnight.

Prepare and preheat barbecue to high heat. Place steaks directly on grill and sear one side for about 15 seconds. Turn steaks over and cook for about 5 minutes, then turn over and cook for another 5 minutes for medium-rare, depending on thickness. Test for doneness by cutting into the middle of the steak.

Dad's Steak Rub

Ingredients

4 beef steaks
1/4 cup maple syrup
1 tablespoon crushed garlic
1 tablespoon seasoned salt
1 tablespoon ground black pepper

Directions

Preheat the grill for high heat.

Place the steaks in a bowl, and drizzle on both sides with maple syrup. Rub with garlic, seasoned salt, and pepper.

Lightly oil the grill grate. Place steaks on the grill, and cook 7 minutes per side, or to desired doneness.

Chicken Fried Venison Steaks

Ingredients

1 egg
1 cup whole milk
2 tablespoons hot pepper sauce
2 pounds 1/2 inch thick venison steaks

1/2 cup cornmeal
1/2 cup seasoned bread crumbs
1 teaspoon cornstarch
1 teaspoon baking soda
1 teaspoon ground black pepper
1 teaspoon garlic salt

1 cup vegetable oil for frying
1 onion, sliced
1 cup whole milk

Directions

Beat the egg in a bowl, then whisk in 1 cup of milk and the hot pepper sauce. Pound the venison steaks with a meat mallet to 1/4 inch thick, and place into the milk mixture. Stir together the cornmeal, bread crumbs, cornstarch, baking soda, black pepper, and garlic salt in a shallow dish.

Remove the venison steaks from the milk mixture one at a time, allowing the excess to run off, and press into the bread crumb mixture; set aside. Reserve the remaining bread crumb mixture.

Heat the oil in a large skillet over medium heat. Place as many breaded venison steaks into the pan as will fit without overlapping. Cook until the venison is golden brown on both sides, about 3 minutes per side. Remove to drain on a paper towel lined plate and keep warm. Repeat with remaining venison.

Once the venison has finished cooking, stir the onions into the hot oil, and cook until dark brown, about 5 minutes. Pour off and discard the oil, remove the onions to a plate and set aside. Stir the reserved bread crumb mixture into the hot skillet, and cook for a few seconds until it begins to toast. Stir in the remaining cup of milk, and simmer until the milk has thickened, about 5 minutes. Pour the gravy over the venison steaks and top with the caramelized onions to serve.

Swordfish Steaks with Arugula and Basil Sauce

Ingredients

4 (6 ounce) swordfish steaks
salt and ground black pepper to taste
1/4 cup extra-virgin olive oil
2 cloves garlic, crushed
1 tablespoon chopped fresh parsley
7 fresh basil leaves, chopped
1 bunch arugula, coarsely chopped
2 tablespoons lemon juice

Directions

Wash and pat dry the swordfish steaks; season each with salt and pepper; completely coat each steak with olive oil.

Heat a grill pan over medium heat; cook the steaks in the grill pan for 15 minutes, turning twice.

While the steaks cook, stir together the garlic, parsley, basil, arugula, and lemon juice in a bowl until evenly coated; spoon over the cooked steaks to serve.

Venison Burger and Steak Chili

Ingredients

1/2 pound bulk mild Italian sausage
1 pound cubed lean venison
2 pounds ground venison
2 tablespoons olive oil
8 ounces sliced crimini mushrooms
1 large onion, diced
2 tablespoons minced garlic
1 green pepper, diced
1 red peppers, diced
2 red chile peppers, seeded and chopped
2 jalapeno peppers, seeded and minced
1 (6 ounce) can tomato paste
1 (28 ounce) can tomato sauce
2 (15.5 ounce) cans black beans, rinsed and drained
2 (28 ounce) cans diced tomatoes, with liquid
1 cup water, or as needed
1/4 teaspoon chili powder
2 tablespoons paprika
1 dash cayenne pepper
2 tablespoons dried oregano
Salt and pepper to taste
1/4 cup minced fresh parsley
1 (8 ounce) package shredded Cheddar cheese

Directions

Cook sausage in a large skillet over medium-high heat until crumbled and browned; place into a large Dutch oven. Sear venison cubes until well browned; add to sausage. Add ground venison, and cook until crumbly and no longer pink; place into Dutch oven.

Heat olive oil in the skillet over medium-high heat. Stir in the mushrooms, and cook until soft, about 2 minutes. Stir in onion and garlic, cook until the onion is translucent, about 2 minutes. Add the green and red peppers, red chile pepper, and jalapeno; cook until softened, then add to Dutch oven.

Stir in tomato paste, tomato sauce, black beans, diced tomatoes, and water. Season with chili powder, paprika, cayenne, and oregano. Bring to a simmer over medium-high heat, then reduce heat to medium-low, cover, and simmer until the venison pieces are tender, about 2 hours.

Season to taste with salt and pepper, and stir in parsley before serving. To serve, sprinkle with shredded Cheddar cheese.

Korean Marinated Flank Steak

Ingredients

- 4 cloves garlic
- 1 teaspoon minced fresh ginger
- 1 onion, roughly chopped
- 2 1/2 cups low sodium soy sauce
- 1/4 cup toasted sesame oil
- 3 tablespoons Worcestershire sauce
- 2 tablespoons unseasoned meat tenderizer
- 1 cup white sugar
- 2 pounds beef flank steak, trimmed of excess fat

Directions

Place garlic, ginger, and onion in the bowl of a blender. Add soy sauce, sesame oil, Worcestershire sauce, meat tenderizer, and sugar. Puree until smooth.

Pour the marinade into a resealable plastic bag or glass bowl. Score the flank steak and place into the marinade. Marinate overnight in the refrigerator.

Preheat a grill for medium-high heat.

Grill steak on preheated grill to desired doneness, about 7 minutes per side for medium.

Mushroom Round Steak

Ingredients

1/2 cup all-purpose flour
1 teaspoon salt
1/4 teaspoon pepper
2 pounds boneless beef round steak, cut into serving-size pieces
2 tablespoons vegetable oil
1 (10.5 ounce) can condensed French onion soup, undiluted
1 (8 ounce) can mushroom stems and pieces, drained
3/4 cup water
1/4 cup ketchup
1 tablespoon Worcestershire sauce
2 tablespoons cornstarch
1/4 cup cold water
1 cup sour cream

Directions

In a large resealable plastic bag, combine the flour, salt and pepper. Add beef, a few pieces at a time, and shake to coat. In a large skillet, brown the beef in batches in oil. Transfer meat to a slow cooker with a slotted spoon. In a bowl, combine the soup, mushrooms, water, ketchup and Worcestershire sauce. Pour over meat. Cover and cook on low for 8 hours or until meat is tender.

Remove beef with a slotted spoon; keep warm. Transfer cooking liquid to a saucepan. Combine cornstarch and cold water until smooth; gradually stir into cooking liquid. bring to a boil; cook and store for 1-2 minutes or until thickened. Stir a small amount of hot liquid into sour cream. Return all to the pan; cook on low until heated through. Serve over meat.

Tangy Ham Steak

Ingredients

1/2 cup ketchup
1/3 cup sweet pickle relish
1 tablespoon cider vinegar
1 teaspoon brown sugar
1/8 teaspoon cayenne pepper
1 pound fully cooked ham steak

Directions

In a bowl, combine the ketchup, relish, vinegar, brown sugar and cayenne; set aside 1/2 cup for serving. Grill the ham steak, uncovered, over medium heat for 3 minutes on each side, basting occasionally with remaining sauce. Serve with reserved sauce.

Beer and Brown Sugar Steak Marinade

Ingredients

2 (16 ounce) beef sirloin steaks
1/4 cup dark beer
2 tablespoons teriyaki sauce
2 tablespoons brown sugar
1/2 teaspoon seasoned salt
1/2 teaspoon black pepper
1/2 teaspoon garlic powder

Directions

Preheat grill for high heat.

Use a fork to poke holes all over the surface of the steaks, and place steaks in a large baking dish. In a bowl, mix together beer, teriyaki sauce, and brown sugar. Pour sauce over steaks, and let sit about 5 minutes. Sprinkle with 1/2 the seasoned salt, pepper, and garlic powder; set aside for 10 minutes. Turn steaks over, sprinkle with remaining seasoned salt, pepper, and garlic powder, and continue marinating for 10 more minutes.

Remove steaks from marinade. Pour marinade into a small saucepan, bring to a boil, and cook for several minutes.

Lightly oil the grill grate. Grill steaks for 7 minutes per side, or to desired doneness. During the last few minutes of grilling, baste steaks with boiled marinade to enhance the flavor and ensure juiciness.

Salisbury Steak Deluxe

Ingredients

1 (10.75 ounce) can condensed cream of mushroom soup, undiluted
1 tablespoon prepared mustard
2 teaspoons Worcestershire sauce
1 teaspoon prepared horseradish
1 egg
1/4 cup dry bread crumbs
1/4 cup finely chopped onion
1/2 teaspoon salt
Dash pepper
1 1/2 pounds ground beef
1 tablespoon cooking oil
1/2 cup water
2 tablespoons chopped fresh parsley

Directions

In a bowl, combine the soup, mustard, Worcestershire sauce and horseradish; blend well. Set aside. In another bowl, lightly beat the egg. Add bread crumbs, onion, salt, pepper and 1/4 cup of the soup mixture. Add beef and mix well. Shape into six patties.

In a large skillet, brown the patties in oil; drain. Combine remaining soup mixture with water; pour over patties. Cover and cook over low heat for 10-15 minutes or until meat is done. Remove patties to a serving platter; spoon sauce over meat. Sprinkle with parsley.

Oven-Fried Ranch Steak

Ingredients

1 cup Ranch salad dressing
1 teaspoon Cajun seasoning
3/4 pound boneless beef sirloin steak
1/3 cup cornmeal
1/3 cup dry bread crumbs
1/2 teaspoon garlic powder

Directions

In a large resealable plastic bag, combine salad dressing and seasoning; add the beef. Seal bag and turn to coat; refrigerate for at least 8 hours or overnight. Drain and discard marinade. In a shallow plate, combine the cornmeal, bread crumbs and garlic powder. Coat both sides of beef in cornmeal mixture.

Place in a greased 13-in. x 9-in. x 2-in. baking dish. Bake at 350 degrees F for 30-35 minutes or until a meat reaches desired doneness (for medium-rare, a meat thermometer should read 145 degrees F; medium, 160 degrees F; well-done, 170 degrees F).

Cubed Steak and Wild Rice

Ingredients

2 tablespoons butter
1 pound cube steak, cut into bite size pieces
1 (4.5 ounce) package long grain and wild rice mix
2 cups water
5 fresh mushrooms, sliced
2 tablespoons Worcestershire sauce
2 tablespoons garlic powder
1 tablespoon onion powder

Directions

In a skillet over medium heat, melt the butter, and saute the cube steak until evenly browned.

In a medium pot, mix the cooked steak and juices, rice, water, mushrooms, Worcestershire sauce, garlic powder, and onion powder. Bring to boil. Reduce heat to low, and simmer 25 minutes, or until all liquid has been absorbed.

Cube Steak Parmigiana

Ingredients

3 tablespoons all-purpose flour
1/2 teaspoon salt
1/4 teaspoon pepper
1 egg
1 tablespoon water
1/3 cup grated Parmesan cheese
1/3 cup finely crushed saltines
1/2 teaspoon dried basil
6 (4 ounce) cube steaks
2 tablespoons vegetable oil
SAUCE:
1 (15 ounce) can tomato sauce
1 tablespoon sugar
1 garlic clove, minced
1/2 teaspoon dried oregano, divided
3 slices mozzarella cheese, halved
1/3 cup grated Parmesan cheese

Directions

In three shallow bowls, combine flour, salt and pepper; beat egg and water; and combine Parmesan cheese, saltines and basil. Dip steaks in flour mixture and egg mixture, then roll in cheese mixture.

In a large skillet, heat 1 tablespoon of oil over medium-high heat. Brown three steaks on both sides. Remove to a greased 13-in. x 9-in. x 2-in. baking pan. Repeat with the remaining steaks, adding additional oil as needed. Bake, uncovered, at 375 degrees F for 25 minutes. Drain any pan juices.

Combine the tomato sauce, sugar, garlic and 1/4 teaspoon of oregano; pour over steaks. Bake 20 minutes longer. Place mozzarella cheese on steaks. Sprinkle with Parmesan and remaining oregano. Return to the oven for 5 minutes or until cheese is melted.

Sirloin Steak with Garlic Butter

Ingredients

1/2 cup butter
2 teaspoons garlic powder
4 cloves garlic, minced
4 pounds beef top sirloin steaks
salt and pepper to taste

Directions

Preheat an outdoor grill for high heat.

In a small saucepan, melt butter over medium-low heat with garlic powder and minced garlic. Set aside.

Sprinkle both sides of each steak with salt and pepper.

Grill steaks 4 to 5 minutes per side, or to desired doneness. When done, transfer to warmed plates. Brush tops liberally with garlic butter, and allow to rest for 2 to 3 minutes before serving.

Sweet Grilled Steak Bites

Ingredients

2 pounds cubed beef stew meat
1/2 teaspoon Greek seasoning, or to taste
1/4 cup soy sauce
1/3 cup dark corn syrup
1 teaspoon minced garlic
1/2 teaspoon seasoned salt

Directions

Season the meat with Greek seasoning. In a large resealable bag or non reactive bowl, combine the soy sauce, corn syrup, garlic and seasoned salt. Massage the bag to blend, then add the beef. Press out most of the air and seal. Marinate for up to 24 hours, flipping over occasionally to evenly marinate.

Preheat a grill for medium heat. When hot, lightly oil the grate. Thread the beef cubes onto skewers.

Grill the meat on the preheated grill, turning occasionally, until they have reached your desired degree of doneness. Be careful not to let the flames get too high. These will darken quickly because of the high sugar content. Don't worry- they aren't burning!

Braised Skirt Steak with Artichoke

Ingredients

1 cube beef bouillon
1/2 cup boiling water
2 tablespoons olive oil
1 pound tenderized skirt steak
1 pinch salt
1 cup marinated artichoke hearts, chopped, liquid reserved
1/2 cup roasted red peppers, drained and chopped
2 pickled jalapeno peppers, chopped
1/2 cup pickled carrots, chopped
1 teaspoon capers
2 tablespoons prepared horseradish

Directions

Preheat an oven to 400 degrees F (200 degrees C).

Dissolve beef boullion cube in boiling water. Heat the olive oil in an oven-safe Dutch oven over high heat. Season the skirt steak on both sides with salt, and cook in the hot oil until browned on both sides, about 2 minutes per side.

Pour the beef bouillon and 1/4 cup artichoke juice into the Dutch oven, then stir in the artichokes, red peppers, jalapeno peppers, carrots, capers, and horseradish. Bring to a boil, then cover, and place into the preheated oven. Bake until the meat has turned from red to light pink in the center, about 30 minutes.

Remove the skirt steak from the Dutch oven, cover with foil, and keep warm. Return the Dutch oven to the stove, and simmer, uncovered, over medium-high heat until the sauce has reduced to your desired consistency, about 10 minutes. Slice the skirt steak thinly, and serve with the reduced sauce.

Brandied Pepper Steak

Ingredients

1 (1 1/2 pound) top round steak
2 teaspoons coarse kosher salt
2 tablespoons black peppercorns, coarsely ground
1/2 cup clarified butter, melted
2 leaves fresh sage, bruised
1 sprig fresh thyme, bruised
4 sprigs fresh rosemary, bruised
1/4 cup brandy
1/2 cup veal demi glace
1/2 cup heavy cream
1 tablespoon roux

Directions

Season steak with salt and pepper, and firmly press seasonings into steak. In a large heavy skillet over medium heat, combine clarified butter, sage, thyme and rosemary. Cook until herbs begin to brown, then remove herbs.

Increase heat to medium-high. Sear steak for 10 to 15 minutes on each side. Carefully pour brandy over steak. Stand back, and ignite the brandy (flames can be quite intense). When flames die, remove steak from pan; keep warm.

Stir demi glace into pan, and deglaze the pan, scraping up any bits stuck to the bottom. Simmer until liquid is reduced by half. Stir in heavy cream, and any juices that have accumulated under the steak. Add roux to sauce to thicken to a smooth, rich consistency. Taste sauce and add more peppercorns or salt if desired.

Chicken Pepper Steak

Ingredients

1 tablespoon vegetable oil
4 boneless, skinless chicken breasts
1 teaspoon seasoning salt
1/2 teaspoon onion powder
2 teaspoons minced garlic
1/2 cup soy sauce, divided
1 large onion, cut into long slices
2 tablespoons cornstarch
2 1/2 cups water
1 green bell pepper, sliced
4 roma (plum) tomatoes, seeded and chopped

Directions

Heat oil in a large skillet over medium heat. Season chicken with salt and onion powder, and place in skillet. Cook for about 5 to 7 minutes, then add the garlic, 4 tablespoons soy sauce, and half of the sliced onion. Cook until chicken is no longer pink, and the juices run clear.

Dissolve cornstarch in water in a small bowl, and blend into the chicken mixture. Stir in 4 tablespoons soy sauce, bell pepper, tomatoes, and remaining onion. Simmer until gravy has reached desired consistency.

Salisbury Steak

Ingredients

1 (10.5 ounce) can condensed French onion soup
1 1/2 pounds ground beef
1/2 cup dry bread crumbs
1 egg
1/4 teaspoon salt
1/8 teaspoon ground black pepper
1 tablespoon all-purpose flour
1/4 cup ketchup
1/4 cup water
1 tablespoon Worcestershire sauce
1/2 teaspoon mustard powder

Directions

In a large bowl, mix together 1/3 cup condensed French onion soup with ground beef, bread crumbs, egg, salt and black pepper. Shape into 6 oval patties.

In a large skillet over medium-high heat, brown both sides of patties. Pour off excess fat.

In a small bowl, blend flour and remaining soup until smooth. Mix in ketchup, water, Worcestershire sauce and mustard powder. Pour over meat in skillet. Cover, and cook for 20 minutes, stirring occasionally.

Steak Salad (Ranen Salad)

Ingredients

1 1/2 pounds beef sirloin steak
8 cups romaine lettuce, torn into bite-size pieces
6 roma (plum) tomatoes, sliced 1/2 cup sliced fresh mushrooms 3/4 cup crumbled blue cheese 1/4 cup walnuts

1/3 cup vegetable oil
3 tablespoons red wine vinegar
2 tablespoons lemon juice
1/2 teaspoon salt
1/8 teaspoon ground black pepper
3 teaspoons Worcestershire sauce
1/8 teaspoon liquid smoke flavoring

Directions

Preheat oven on broiler setting. Broil steaks for 3 to 5 minutes per side, or to desired doneness. Allow to cool, then slice into bite-size pieces.

On chilled plates, arrange lettuce, tomatoes, and mushrooms. Sprinkle with blue cheese and walnuts. Top with steak slices.

In a small bowl, whisk together oil, vinegar, lemon juice, salt, pepper, Worcestershire sauce, and smoke flavoring. Drizzle over salad.

Easy Minute Steaks

Ingredients

4 (1/2 pound) cube steaks (pounded round meat)
1 (10.5 ounce) can condensed French onion soup

Directions

Preheat oven to 350 degrees F (175 degrees C).

In a large skillet over medium heat, briefly brown the cube steaks.

Arrange meat in a single layer in a 13x9 inch baking dish and pour the soup over the top. Bake in preheated oven for 1 hour.

Steak Burritos

Ingredients

2 flank steaks (1 pound each)
2 (1.25 ounce) packages taco seasoning
1 medium onion, chopped
1 (4 ounce) can chopped green chilies
1 tablespoon vinegar
10 (8 inch) flour tortillas
1 1/2 cups shredded Monterey Jack cheese
1 1/2 cups chopped, seeded plum tomatoes
3/4 cup sour cream

Directions

Cut steaks in half; rub with taco seasoning. Place in a slow cooker coated with nonstick cooking spray. Top with onion, chilies and vinegar. Cover and cook on low for 8-9 hours or until meat is tender. Remove steaks and cool slightly; shred meat with two forks. (Turn to page 51 for a tip on shredding meat.) Return to slow cooker; heat through. Spoon about 1/2 cup meat mixture down the center of each tortilla. Top with cheese, tomato and sour cream. Fold ends and sides over filling.

Chicken Fried Steak III

Ingredients

2 1/2 cups all-purpose flour, divided
2 tablespoons salt
1 teaspoon cayenne pepper
3 eggs, lightly beaten
3 pounds beef chuck steaks, well trimmed
1 cup oil for frying
2 1/2 cups milk
1 teaspoon garlic salt
3/4 teaspoon celery salt
2 tablespoons chili powder
1 cube beef bouillon

Directions

In a shallow bowl, combine 2 cups of the flour, salt and cayenne pepper; set aside. In a bowl, beat together eggs and remaining 1/2 cup flour. Pound steaks flat with a meat mallet. Dredge the steaks first in the flour mixture, then into the egg mixture, then back into the flour mixture.

Heat oil in a large skillet over medium high heat. Fry the coated steaks until golden brown. Remove from skillet, drain, and keep warm.

Pour off all but 1 tablespoon of the oil, then stir in the leftover seasoned flour. Cook over medium heat, stirring constantly, until the flour is browned. Remove from the heat and Stir in milk, garlic salt, celery salt, chili powder and beef bouillon. Return to the heat and bring to a simmer, stirring constantly, until gravy thickens.

Chinese Pepper Steak

Ingredients

1 1/2 cups julienned green bell pepper
3/4 cup chopped onion
2 tablespoons vegetable oil, divided
2 cups sliced fresh mushrooms
3/4 pound boneless beef sirloin steak, cut into thin strips
1/2 teaspoon salt
1/4 teaspoon pepper
1 clove garlic, minced
1 tablespoon cornstarch
1 cup apple juice
1/4 cup cold water
Hot cooked rice

Directions

In a wok or skillet, stir-fry green peppers and onion in 1 tablespoon oil for 2-3 minutes. Add mushrooms; stir-fry 1 minute longer. Remove and keep warm.

Season the beef with salt and pepper. In the same skillet, stir-fry the beef and garlic in remaining oil for 6-8 minutes or until no longer pink; drain.

Combine the cornstarch, apple juice and water until smooth; stir into the beef mixture. Bring to a boil; cook and stir for 1 minutes or until thickened. Return the vegetables to the pan; heat through.
Serve over the rice.

Teriyaki Rib Eye Steaks

Ingredients

2 tablespoons soy sauce
2 tablespoons water
1 tablespoon white sugar
1 1/2 teaspoons honey
1 1/2 teaspoons Worcestershire sauce
1 1/4 teaspoons distilled white vinegar
1 teaspoon olive oil
1/4 teaspoon onion powder
1/4 teaspoon garlic powder
1/8 teaspoon ground ginger
2 (6 ounce) lean beef rib eye steaks

Directions

Whisk together the soy sauce, water, sugar, honey, Worcestershire sauce, vinegar, olive oil, onion powder, garlic powder, and ground ginger in a large bowl. Pierce steaks several times with a fork. Marinate steaks in soy sauce mixture for at least 2 hours.

Cook the steaks in a hot skillet, wok, or hibachi over medium heat; 7 minutes per side for medium. An instant-read thermometer inserted into the center should read 140 degrees F (60 degrees C).

Steak 'N' Vegetable Soup

Ingredients

1 pound boneless beef sirloin steak, cut into 1/2 inch cubes
1 cup chopped onion
2 teaspoons canola oil
2 cups cubed red potatoes
1 cup chopped carrots
1 cup frozen peas
1 (14.5 ounce) can beef broth
1 cup water
2 tablespoons balsamic vinegar
1 tablespoon minced fresh parsley
1 tablespoon minced chives
1 1/2 teaspoons minced fresh basil
1 teaspoon minced fresh thyme
3/4 teaspoon salt
1/4 teaspoon pepper

Directions

In a large saucepan, cook beef and onion in oil until meat is no longer pink; drain. Stir in the potatoes, carrots and peas. Add the broth, water, vinegar, parsley, chives, basil, thyme, salt and pepper. Bring to a boil. Reduce heat; cover and simmer for 20-30 minutes or until meat and vegetables are tender.

Peppered Steak with Blackberry Sauce

Ingredients

1/3 cup lemon juice
1/3 cup Crisco® Vegetable Oil
1/4 cup chopped onion
2 cloves garlic, minced
4 (4 ounce) beef tenderloin or eye of round steaks, trimmed of fat
Salt and coarsely ground black pepper
Crisco® Original No-Stick Cooking Spray
1/2 cup Smucker's® Seedless Blackberry Jam
1/4 cup red wine vinegar
1/4 teaspoon onion powder
1/4 cup fresh or thawed frozen blackberries

Directions

Mix lemon juice, oil, onion and garlic in large re-sealable plastic bag. Place steaks in marinade. Seal bag and refrigerate 6 to 24 hours, turning bag occasionally. When ready to cook, season steaks with salt and coarsely ground pepper. Discard marinade.

Spray grill rack with no-stick cooking spray. Heat grill.

Cook jam, vinegar and onion powder in small saucepan over medium heat until jam is melted, stirring constantly. Remove from heat.

Place steaks on prepared grill. Cook 8 to 12 minutes or until desired doneness, turning once halfway through cooking time. To serve, top steaks with blackberry sauce. Sprinkle with fresh blackberries.

Wasabi Encrusted Tuna Steaks

Ingredients

1 tablespoon five-spice powder
1 tablespoon grated fresh ginger
2 tablespoons sake
2 tablespoons rice vinegar
2 tablespoons tamari
1/4 cup sesame oil
2 pounds ahi tuna steaks, each about 1 inch thick
1 pound wasabi peas, crushed
2 tablespoons light brown sugar

Directions

In a large bowl, whisk together the five-spice powder, ginger, sake, rice vinegar, tamari, and sesame oil. Add the tuna steaks and turn to coat; allow to marinate for 30 minutes.

Combine the crushed wasabi peas and brown sugar. Remove the tuna steaks from the marinade, and press into the pea mixture to coat. Pour the marinade into a small saucepan and bring to a simmer over medium-high heat. Reduce heat to medium, and simmer until the sauce has reduced and thickened, 5 to 10 minutes.

While the sauce is cooking, sear the tuna in a small amount of oil in a skillet over medium-high heat to desired doneness. Pour sauce over tuna to serve.

Grilled Salmon Steaks Italian-Style

Ingredients

2 salmon steaks
1 tablespoon dried Italian seasoning
1 teaspoon crumbled dried thyme
1 teaspoon crushed dried rosemary
salt and pepper to taste
1 tablespoon fresh lime juice

Directions

Preheat an outdoor grill for medium heat and lightly oil grate.

Season one side of each steak with the Italian seasoning, thyme, rosemary, salt, and pepper.

Lay the steaks with the seasoned-side down on the prepared grill. Cook on grill until the flesh flakes, turning once, 7 to 8 minutes. Sprinkle each steak with lime juice to serve.

Paprika Chili Steak

Ingredients

- 1 medium onion, chopped
- 1/2 cup ketchup
- 1/4 cup cider vinegar
- 1 tablespoon paprika
- 1 tablespoon canola oil
- 2 teaspoons chili powder
- 1 teaspoon salt
- 1/8 teaspoon pepper
- 1 1/2 pounds beef flank steak

Directions

In a large resealable plastic bag, combine the first eight ingredients; add steak. Seal bag and turn to coat; refrigerate for 3 hours or overnight, turning occasionally.

Coat grill rack with nonstick cooking spray before starting the grill. Drain and discard marinade. Grill steak, covered, over medium-hot heat for 6-8 minutes on each side or until meat reaches desired doneness (for medium-rare, a meat thermometer should read 145 degrees F; medium, 160 degrees F, well-done, 170 degrees F.

Steak House Au Gratin Potatoes

Ingredients

1 tablespoon butter
3 russet potato, peeled and cubed
1 cup heavy cream
1/2 cup 2% reduced-fat milk
4 cloves garlic, minced
2 tablespoons all-purpose flour
salt and black pepper to taste
1 cup grated medium Cheddar cheese

Directions

Preheat an oven to 350 degrees F (175 degrees C). Grease one 9x13 inch baking pan with butter. Spread potatoes evenly in the pan.

Whisk together heavy cream, milk, garlic, flour, salt, and pepper in a large bowl. Pour cream mixture over the potatoes. Cover with foil.

Bake in the preheated oven for 20 minutes, then remove the foil. Continue baking until the potatoes are easily pierced with a fork, about 40 minutes. Remove potatoes from the oven and sprinkle Cheddar cheese on top. Return to oven and bake until the cheese is melted, 5 to 10 minutes. Allow to cool for 5 minutes before serving.

Thyme-Rubbed Steaks with Sauteed Mushrooms

Ingredients

2 teaspoons paprika
1 teaspoon salt
1 teaspoon ground black pepper
1/2 teaspoon garlic powder
1/2 teaspoon onion powder
1/2 teaspoon dried thyme

1 pound New York strip steaks, cut 3/4 inch thick
1 (8 ounce) package sliced fresh mushrooms
1/4 cup minced shallot
2 tablespoons butter
2 tablespoons red wine
1 tablespoon vegetable oil
salt and pepper to taste

Directions

In a small bowl, mix together the paprika, salt, pepper, garlic powder, onion powder and thyme. Sprinkle onto each side of the steaks, pressing in so it adheres. Set aside.

Melt the butter in a skillet over medium-high heat. Add the shallots; cook and stir for about 1 minute. Add the mushrooms, and cook for a few more minutes, until tender. Stir in the red wine, and cook until most of the liquid has evaporated. Remove from the heat and keep warm.

Heat the oil in a separate skillet over medium-high heat. Fry steaks for 5 to 7 minutes per side, or to your desired degree of doneness. Remove to a plate and let rest for a few minutes. Top with mushrooms and serve.

Spicy Lime-Cilantro Marinated Flank Steak

Ingredients

6 cloves garlic
1/2 red onion, chopped
2 limes, juiced
1 medium jalapeno chile pepper
2 tablespoons fresh thyme leaves
1 cup loosely packed cilantro leaves
3/4 cup corn oil
2 tablespoons honey
3 pounds beef flank steak
kosher salt to taste

Directions

Puree the garlic, onion, lime juice, jalapeno, thyme, cilantro, corn oil, and honey into the bowl of a blender or food processor until the ingredients are well incorporated. Marinate the flank steak with 1/2 cup of the puree in a resealable bag overnight in the refrigerator. Reserve the rest of the puree to use later as a sauce.

Preheat a grill for medium-high heat.

While grill is warming, remove the meat from the refrigerator and let sit at room temperature for at least 30 minutes. Discard any marinade left in the bag. Liberally season the steak with the kosher salt, and cook to desired doneness, approximately 4 minutes per side for medium-rare.

To serve, slice the steak against the grain into 1/8 to 1/4 inch slices, and drizzle the remaining marinade over the meat.

Peanut Sesame Rib-Eye Steak

Ingredients

4 stalks lemon grass, coarsely chopped
1/4 cup vegetable oil
1/4 cup fish sauce
1/4 cup rice wine vinegar
1 teaspoon dark soy sauce
1 teaspoon white sugar
1/2 teaspoon Asian (toasted) sesame oil

4 (8 ounce) beef rib eye steaks (thick-cut)

1/2 cup chopped peanuts 1/2 cup black sesame seeds 1/4 cup sea salt
1/4 cup crushed black peppercorns

1 tablespoon vegetable oil, divided

Directions

Place the lemon grass, 1/4 cup vegetable oil, fish sauce, rice wine vinegar, dark soy sauce, sugar, and sesame oil into the work bowl of a food processor, and process until the mixture forms a paste. Coat both sides of the steaks with the marinade paste, and refrigerate, covered, for 2 to 3 hours.

Preheat an outdoor grill for medium-high heat, and lightly oil the grate.

In a bowl, combine peanuts, sesame seeds, sea salt, and pepper until thoroughly mixed.

Remove the steaks from the marinade, and discard any remaining marinade. Pat the steaks very dry with paper towels for good charring. Rub each steak with about 3/4 teaspoon of vegetable oil. Sprinkle the peanut mixture generously over both sides of each steak, and press the spices into the meat.

Grill on the preheated grill until the steaks show grill marks, start to become firm, and are reddish-pink and juicy in the center, 4 to 5 minutes per side. An instant-read thermometer inserted into the center should read 130 degrees F (54 degrees C). Let the steaks rest at least 5 minutes before slicing.

Ostrich Steaks with Calvados Sauce

Ingredients

2 tablespoons clarified butter
4 (5 ounce) ostrich steaks
1/2 cup beef stock
1/3 cup creme fraiche
1/4 cup Calvados (apple brandy)
salt and ground black pepper to taste

Directions

Heat the butter in a skillet over medium-high heat. Cook the ostrich steaks in the hot butter until the outside is just about to be crisp, shown by darkening patches as with a beef steak, about 2 minutes per side. An instant-read thermometer inserted into the center should read 145 degrees F (63 degrees C) for rare. Remove the ostrich steaks from the pan, and keep warm.

Pour the beef stock into the skillet, and bring to a boil over high heat. Boil for a few minutes until slightly reduced, then lower the heat to medium-low, and stir in the creme fraiche. Cook and stir 2 minutes, then pour in the Calvados, and season to taste with salt and pepper. Season each ostrich steak with pepper to taste. Spoon the sauce over the steaks to serve.

Willy's Juicy Steak

Ingredients

2 cups orange juice
1 cup thousand island salad dressing
1 cup Worcestershire sauce
2 tablespoons vinegar-based hot pepper sauce
2 tablespoons minced fresh garlic
4 (1/2 pound) 1 1/2 inch thick rib-eye steaks
salt and pepper to taste

Directions

In a large resealable plastic bag, combine the orange juice, salad dressing, Worcestershire sauce, hot pepper sauce, and garlic. Squeeze the bag to mix well. You should have a nice brown marinade. Place steaks into the bag with the marinade, and seal. Refrigerate for 2 to 5 hours, turning over occasionally.

Preheat an outdoor grill for high heat. When the grill is hot, lightly oil the grate.

Place steaks onto the grill and season the tops with salt and pepper to taste. Baste with marinade. Cook for about 5 to 7 minutes, then flip over and salt, pepper and baste again. Grill for about 7 or 8 more minutes, or to desired doneness. Do not flip the steaks again. The internal temperature should be at least 145 degrees F (63 degrees C). Let steaks stand for 5 minutes before cutting, to prevent juices from running out.

Heat the remaining marinade to a boil in a small saucepan. Use as steak sauce.

Flank Steak Pinwheels

Ingredients

1/4 cup olive oil
1/4 cup soy sauce
1/4 cup red wine
1/4 cup Worcestershire sauce
1 tablespoon Dijon mustard
1 tablespoon lemon juice
1 clove garlic, minced
1 teaspoon Italian seasoning
1/2 teaspoon ground black pepper

1 1/2 pounds flank steak, pounded to 1/2 inch thickness

1 clove garlic, peeled
1/4 teaspoon salt
1/4 cup chopped onion
1/4 cup fine dry bread crumbs
1 cup frozen chopped spinach, thawed and squeezed dry
1/2 cup crumbled feta cheese

Directions

In a large resealable bag, combine the olive oil, soy sauce, red wine, Worcestershire sauce, mustard, lemon juice, 1 clove of garlic, Italian seasoning and pepper. Squeeze the bag to blend well. Pierce the flank steak with a knife, making small slits about 1 inch apart. Place the steak into the bag, and seal. Refrigerate overnight to marinate.

Preheat the oven to 350 degrees F (175 degrees C).

Crush the remaining clove of garlic on a cutting board with a large chef's knife. Sprinkle the salt over the garlic, and scrape with the blunt side of the knife to make a paste.

Remove the steak from the bag, and discard marinade. Spread the garlic paste over the top side of the steak. Place layers of chopped onion, bread crumbs, spinach, and cheese over the garlic. Roll the steak up lengthwise, and secure with kitchen twine or toothpicks. Place the roll in a shallow glass baking dish.

Bake uncovered for 1 hour in the preheated oven, or until the internal temperature of the roll is at least 145 degrees F (63 degrees F) in the center. Let stand for 5 minutes to set, then slice into 1 inch slices to serve.

Japanese Sesame Steak Sauce

Ingredients

1/4 cup tahini
2 tablespoons soy sauce
1 tablespoon mayonnaise
1 clove garlic, minced
1 1/2 teaspoons ground ginger
1 pinch paprika
1/4 cup water, or as needed

Directions

Whisk the tahini, soy sauce, mayonnaise, garlic, ginger, and paprika together in a bowl. Gradually stir the water into the mixture until you reach a desired consistency. Refrigerate until ready to use.

Luau Beef Tenderloin Steaks

Ingredients

- 1/4 cup unsweetened pineapple juice
- 1/4 cup reduced-sodium soy sauce
- 1/4 cup olive oil
- 2 tablespoons lemon juice
- 2 tablespoons cider vinegar
- 6 garlic cloves, minced
- 1 tablespoon chopped sweet onion
- 1 1/2 teaspoons ground mustard
- 1/2 teaspoon minced fresh parsley
- 4 (4 ounce) beef tenderloin steaks

Directions

In a small bowl, combine the first nine ingredients. Pour 3/4 cup marinade into a large resealable plastic bag; add the steaks. Seal bag and turn to coat; refrigerate for several hours or overnight. Cover and refrigerate remaining marinade.

Drain steaks and discard marinade. Coat grill rack with nonstick cooking spray before starting the grill. Grill steaks, covered, over medium heat for 6-8 minutes on each side or until meat reaches desired doneness (for medium-rare, a meat thermometer should read 145 degrees F; medium, 160 degrees F; well-done, 170 degrees F). Baste with reserved marinade during the last 2 minutes of cooking.

Bangin' Steak Rub

Ingredients

1/2 cup packed brown sugar
1 (1.25 ounce) package chili seasoning mix
1 (1 ounce) envelope ranch dressing mix
1 teaspoon garlic salt
1 teaspoon onion salt
1/2 teaspoon ground black pepper
1 teaspoon steak seasoning

Directions

In a small bowl, thoroughly mix together the brown sugar, chili seasoning mix, ranch dressing mix, garlic salt, onion salt, ground black pepper, and steak seasoning. The rub should be smooth and granular, with no large lumps. Store at room temperature in an airtight container until ready to use.

To use, rub the seasoning mix liberally onto the steak or meat of your choice before cooking.

Creamy Sliced Steak and Potatoes

Ingredients

1 1/2 teaspoons vegetable oil
1/2 slice onion, diced
14 ounces beef top sirloin, thinly sliced
1 (15 ounce) can whole new potatoes, drained
1 (10.75 ounce) can condensed cream of mushroom soup
1/4 cup milk
salt and pepper to taste

Directions

Heat the vegetable oil in a skillet over medium heat. Stir in the onions, and cook until they begin to soften, about 3 minutes. Increase the heat to medium-high, and add the sliced sirloin. Cook and stir until the meat is no longer pink, and beginning to brown around the edges, about 7 minutes. Add the potatoes, cream of mushroom soup, and milk. Bring to a simmer, then reduce the heat to medium-low, and simmer 10 minutes. Season to taste with salt and pepper before serving.

Flat Iron Steak with Mushrooms

Ingredients

3 tablespoons vegetable oil
salt and pepper to taste
3 (6 ounce) beef flat iron steaks (shoulder top blade)
3 shallots, thinly sliced
6 cloves garlic, peeled
4 cups sliced white mushrooms
1/4 cup balsamic vinegar
3/4 cup full-bodied red wine

Directions

Preheat the oven to 350 degrees F (175 degrees C).

Heat the oil in a large skillet over medium heat. Cut the flat iron steak into individual portions if needed. Season with salt and pepper on both sides. Fry the steaks until browned on each side, 2 to 3 minutes per side. Remove from the skillet and place in an oven proof dish. Set steaks in the oven to continue cooking.

Add shallots and whole cloves of garlic to the hot skillet. Cook and stir over medium heat until shallots are starting to brown. Add mushrooms to the pan; cook and stir until they shrink some, 5 to 10 minutes.

Pour the balsamic vinegar into the pan with the mushrooms and stir to remove any bits that are stuck to the bottom of the skillet. Pour in the red wine and simmer for a few minutes over medium heat.

Return the steaks to the skillet and cook until the internal temperature reaches 135 degrees to 140 degrees F (60 degrees C), about 5 minutes if at all. Remove the whole pan from the heat and let stand until steaks reach an internal temperature of 145 degrees F (63 degrees C), or your desired degree of doneness.

Salsa Steak For One

Ingredients

1 (6 ounce) boneless beef top sirloin steak, cut 1 1/2 inches thick
seasoned salt to taste
3 tablespoons water
1 cup prepared salsa
1 large potato, peeled and diced
1 carrot, peeled and chopped
1 small white onion, diced

Directions

Preheat oven to 350 degrees F (175 degrees C).

Sprinkle both sides of steak with seasoned salt. Place in a foil-lined baking dish with 3 tablespoons of water. Pour salsa over steak, and spread chopped vegetables all around pan. Cover, and seal with foil.

Bake in the preheated oven for one hour, or to desired doneness. Serve immediately.

Pork Steaks

Ingredients

1/4 cup butter
1/4 cup soy sauce
1 bunch green onions
2 cloves garlic, minced
5 pork butt steaks

Directions

Melt butter in a skillet, and mix in the soy sauce. Saute the green onions and garlic until lightly browned.

Place the pork steaks in the skillet, cover, and cook 8 to 10 minutes on each side, Remove cover, and continue cooking 10 minutes, or to an internal temperature of 160 degrees F (70 degrees C).

Steak and Rice

Ingredients

1 1/2 pounds round steak
2 tablespoons vegetable oil
1 green bell pepper
1 (29 ounce) can diced tomatoes
4 tablespoons cornstarch
1 cube beef bouillon cube
1/4 cup soy sauce
1/2 teaspoon garlic powder
1/2 teaspoon ground black pepper
1/2 teaspoon ground ginger
2 cups water

1 cup white rice
2 cups water

Directions

Trim any fat from round steak and slice meat into thin 2 to 3 inch long strips. Remove the seeds and core from the green bell pepper, and slice into thin 3 inch long strips.

In a large frying pan over medium to high heat add oil and cook meat until medium rare, add peppers and continue cooking until meat is browned.

Reduce heat to simmer and add tomatoes, soy sauce, garlic powder, black pepper and ginger. Cover and simmer 10 minutes.

Dissolve bullion cube and corn starch in 2 cups water and stir well before adding to simmering beef. Cover and simmer 10 minutes, stirring occasionally, until sauce resembles the consistency of gravy. Remove from heat and serve over a bed of rice.

To cook rice: In a saucepan, bring 2 cups of water to a boil. Stir in 1 cup of rice. Cover and reduce heat to a simmer. Simmer for 20 minutes.

Flat Iron Steak and Spinach Salad

Ingredients

2 pounds flat iron steak
salt and ground black pepper to taste
2 tablespoons olive oil
1 large red onion, thinly sliced
1/2 cup Italian salad dressing
3 large red bell peppers, cut into 1/2 inch strips
2 portobello mushrooms, sliced
1/2 cup red wine
4 cups baby spinach leaves
1/2 cup crumbled blue cheese

Directions

Preheat an outdoor grill for medium-high heat; lightly oil the grate.

Season the flat iron steak on both sides with salt and pepper. Cook to desired degree of doneness on preheated grill, about 5 minutes per side for medium-rare. Let rest in a warm area while proceeding with the recipe.

Heat olive oil in a large skillet over medium-high heat. Stir in the onion, and cook until it begins to soften, about 4 minutes. Pour in the Italian salad dressing, and bring to a boil, then stir in the red peppers and mushrooms. Reduce heat to medium, and cook until the peppers are tender, about 5 minutes.

Remove the vegetables from the skillet with a slotted spoon, and set aside. Increase the heat to medium-high, and add the red wine. Simmer the salad dressing and wine until it has reduced to a syrupy sauce, about 5 minutes.

Meanwhile, divide the spinach leaves onto serving plates. Thinly slice the flat iron steak across the grain. Spoon the warm, cooked vegetable mixture over the spinach leaves, then place the sliced steak on top. Spoon on the reduced red wine sauce, and finally, sprinkle with blue cheese.

Teriyaki Steak

Ingredients

2 pounds beef skirt steak
4 cloves garlic, minced
2 cups teriyaki sauce

Directions

Cut the skirt steak into individual strips for serving. Add the garlic to the teriyaki sauce. In a re-sealable plastic bag, combine the steak and the sauce. Seal tightly and refrigerate to marinate overnight.

Preheat oven to broil OR preheat a barbecue grill.

When oven OR grill is ready, remove meat from bag and discard remaining marinade. Place meat on a broiler pan for the oven OR directly on the grill for the barbecue. Cook for about 5 minutes per side, or to desired doneness.

Berdean's Cube Steak

Ingredients

4 (4 ounce) cube steaks
salt and pepper to taste
1/4 cup all-purpose flour
1/3 cup vegetable oil
1 teaspoon beef bouillon granules

Directions

Season the cube steaks on both sides with salt and pepper. Pour the flour onto a shallow plate and press the steaks into the flour; shake off the excess flour. Heat the oil in a large skillet with lid over medium-high heat. Place the steaks into the hot oil, and cook until golden brown on both sides, about 3 minutes per side.

Pour water into the skillet to almost cover the steaks. Stir the beef bouillon and salt to taste into the water. Bring to a boil; reduce heat to medium-low, cover, and simmer until very tender, about 2 hours.

Finger Steaks

Ingredients

1 cup all-purpose flour
3 1/2 teaspoons seasoned salt
1 teaspoon ground black pepper

1 egg
1/4 cup buttermilk
1/4 cup dark beer
1 tablespoon hot pepper sauce (such as Frank's RedHot®)

2 pounds flat iron steaks
1 teaspoon seasoned salt

4 cups vegetable oil for frying

Directions

Whisk the flour, 3 1/2 teaspoons seasoned salt, and black pepper together in a mixing bowl; set aside. Beat the egg in a separate mixing bowl, then mix in the buttermilk, beer, and hot pepper sauce until smooth; set aside. Cut the steak into strips 1/2-inch wide by 3- to 4-inches long. Place into a mixing bowl, and toss with the remaining 1 teaspoon of seasoned salt.

Gently press the steak strips into the flour to coat and shake off the excess flour. Place the steak strips into the beaten egg, then toss in the flour again. Gently toss the strips between your hands so the excess flour can fall away. Place onto a baking sheet, and freeze until solid, about 4 hours.

Heat oil in a deep-fryer or large saucepan to 350 degrees F (175 degrees C).

Fry the frozen steak strips in small batches (5 to 7 at a time) until the breading is golden brown, and the beef has cooked to your desired degree of doneness, about 5 minutes for medium-well.

Stir-Fried Steak and Veggies

Ingredients

1 tablespoon cornstarch
1 tablespoon brown sugar
3/4 teaspoon ground ginger
1/2 teaspoon chili powder
1/4 teaspoon garlic powder
1/4 teaspoon pepper
1/2 cup cold water
1/4 cup soy sauce
1 pound boneless sirloin steak, cut into thin strips
2 tablespoons vegetable oil
2 cups broccoli florets
2 cups cauliflowerets
1 large onion, chopped
1 cup sliced carrots
Hot cooked rice

Directions

In a small bowl, whisk together the first eight ingredients until smooth; set aside.

In a skillet or wok, stir-fry steak in oil for 3-5 minutes. Add broccoli, cauliflower, onion, carrots and soy sauce mixture; cover and cook for 8 minutes or until vegetables are crisp-tender, stirring occasionally. Serve over rice.

Pineapple-Green Onion Salsa with Cook's Ham

Ingredients

1 (2 pound) Cook's® brand Bone-in Ham Steaks
2 cups fresh ripe pineapple, trimmed, cored and chopped into 3/8-inch to 1/2-inch chunks
1/4 cup fresh lemon juice, with pulp
1 green onion, minced
1/2 red bell pepper, cored and minced, 1/8-inch to 1/4-inch
1 teaspoon lemon zest, finely minced
3 dashes Tabasco sauce
3/4 teaspoon kosher salt
2 tablespoons brown sugar
1/4 teaspoon dry mustard
1 pinch ground cloves

Directions

Prepare charcoal or gas grill. Place ham steaks on grill over medium-high heat. Grill ham steaks 3 to 5 minutes per side, turning once.

Mix together all ingredients for salsa.

Serve Ham Steak with a side of Pineapple-Green Onion Salsa.

Philly Steak Salad

Ingredients

16 ounces flank steak, cut into strips
1 green bell pepper, seeded and cut into strips
1 large onion, sliced into rings
1 (8 ounce) bottle Italian-style salad dressing
1/2 (32 ounce) package frozen curly-style French fries
1 (8 ounce) package shredded Cheddar cheese
1 head iceberg lettuce, torn into bite-sized pieces
4 tomatoes, quartered
1 (15 ounce) can garbanzo beans, drained
1 (8 ounce) bottle Ranch-style salad dressing

Directions

In a covered dish, spread out sliced steak, peppers and onions and pour the Italian dressing over all. Cover and refrigerate for at least 20 minutes.

Cook French fries according to package instructions while steak is marinating.

In a large skillet over medium-high heat, saute steak, peppers and onions until vegetables are tender and steak is cooked to your liking. Separate steak mixture into 8 equal portions while in the skillet, and top each portion with cheese. Cover and set aside to let cheese melt.

Arrange lettuce, tomatoes and garbanzo beans on 8 separate plates. Top each salad with 1/8 of the French fries and 1/8 of the steak mixture and serve with Ranch-style salad dressing.

Beef Pepper Steak

Ingredients

12 black peppercorns, coarsely ground
2 tablespoons tamari
1 clove garlic, minced
1 pinch white sugar
1 pinch salt
10 ounces beef filet
2 tablespoons butter

Directions

In a small, nonporous bowl, combine the peppercorns, tamari, garlic, sugar and salt. Add the beef filet and coat well on all sides. Cover and marinate in the refrigerator for 1 hour.

Melt butter in a medium saucepan over medium high heat. Place the beef filet in the pan and saute for 6 to 8 minutes per side, or until internal temperature reaches at least 145 degrees F (65 degrees C).

Flash-In-The-Pan Pepper Steak

Ingredients

3/4 pound boneless beef round steak, cut into thin strips
1/2 medium onion, cut into thin wedges
1/2 small green bell pepper, julienned
2 garlic cloves, minced
1 tablespoon butter or margarine
3/4 cup beef broth
1 tablespoon soy sauce
1 tablespoon cornstarch
2 tablespoons cold water
1/2 medium tomato, cut into wedges
1/4 cup fresh or frozen snow peas
1 teaspoon paprika
Hot cooked rice

Directions

In a large skillet, cook the beef, onion, green pepper and garlic in butter over medium heat for 5-7 minutes or until vegetables are tender and meat is no longer pink. Add the broth and soy sauce; bring mixture to a boil. Reduce heat; simmer, uncovered, for 1-2 minutes.

In a small bowl, combine cornstarch and water until smooth; stir into skillet. Bring to a boil; cook and stir for 2 minutes or until thickened. Stir in the tomato, snow peas and paprika; cook 30 seconds longer. Serve over rice.

Marinated Venison Steaks

Ingredients

6 (4 ounce) boneless venison steaks
1/2 cup white vinegar
1/2 cup ketchup
1/4 cup vegetable oil
1/4 cup Worcestershire sauce
4 garlic cloves, minced
1 1/2 teaspoons ground mustard
1/2 teaspoon salt
1/2 teaspoon pepper

Directions

Place venison in a large resealable plastic bag. In a bowl, combine the remaining ingredients. Pour half over the venison; seal bag and turn to coat. Refrigerate overnight. Refrigerate remaining marinade.

Drain and discard marinade from steaks. Broil 3-4 in. from the heat for 4 minutes. Turn; baste with reserved marinade. broil 4 minutes longer, basting often, or until a meat thermometer reads 160 degrees F for medium or 170 degrees F for well-done.

Southwest Steak Bites

Ingredients

1 quart oil for frying
1 egg
1/4 cup milk
2 cups all-purpose flour
2 teaspoons dry mesquite flavored seasoning mix
1 teaspoon salt
1 teaspoon ground black pepper
1/2 teaspoon garlic powder
1/4 teaspoon ground cayenne pepper
2 pounds cube steak, cut into bite size pieces

Directions

Heat the oil in a deep fryer or heavy skillet to 365 degrees F (185 degrees C).

In a bowl, beat together the egg and milk. In a resealable plastic bag, mix the flour, mesquite seasoning, salt, pepper, garlic powder, and cayenne pepper. Dip the steak pieces in the egg mixture, then place in the plastic bag, seal, and shake to coat.

In the hot oil, fry the coated steak pieces in small batches until golden brown, about 5 minutes. Drain on paper towels.

Saskatchewan City Steak Soup

Ingredients

6 tablespoons butter
1/3 cup all-purpose flour
5 cups beef stock
2 beef bouillon cubes
1 cup vegetable juice (such as V8®)
3 dashes Worcestershire sauce
1/2 cup diced celery
1/2 cup peeled, diced carrots
1/2 cup chopped onion
1 head cabbage, shredded
1 (14.5 ounce) can green beans, drained
1 (14.5 ounce) can diced tomatoes
1 pound lean ground beef
1 teaspoon monosodium glutamate (such as Ac'cent®)
1 1/2 teaspoons ground black pepper
1 1/2 teaspoons browning sauce (such as Kitchen Bouquet®)
salt, to taste

Directions

Melt the butter in a large saucepan over medium-low heat. Whisk in the flour, and stir until the mixture becomes paste-like and light golden brown, about 5 minutes. Gradually whisk the beef stock into the flour mixture and bring to a simmer over medium heat. Cook and stir until the mixture is thick and smooth, 10 to 15 minutes. Stir in the bouillon cubes, vegetable juice, and Worcestershire sauce. Bring to a boil over medium-high heat, then add celery, carrots, onion, shredded cabbage, green beans, and tomatoes. Allow soup to return to a boil, then reduce heat to medium-low. Cover and simmer until vegetables are tender, about 30 minutes.

Meanwhile, cook and stir ground beef in a skillet over medium-high heat until browned, about 10 minutes. Drain and set aside. When the vegetables in the soup are tender, stir in the ground beef and simmer for 15 minutes. Stir in monosodium glutamate, pepper, browning sauce, and salt to serve.

Grilled Rib Eye Steaks

Ingredients

1/2 cup soy sauce
1/2 cup sliced green onions
1/4 cup packed brown sugar
2 garlic cloves, minced
1/4 teaspoon ground ginger
1/4 teaspoon pepper
2 1/2 pounds beef rib eye steaks

Directions

In a large resealable plastic bag, combine the soy sauce, onions, brown sugar, garlic, ginger and pepper. Add the steaks. Seal bag and turn to coat; refrigerate for 8 hours or overnight.

Drain and discard marinade. Grill steaks, uncovered, over medium-hot heat for 8-10 minutes or until the meat reaches desired doneness (for medium-rare, a meat thermometer should read 145 degrees F; medium, 160 degrees F; well-done, 170 degrees F).

Bloody Mary Steaks with Green Olive Butter

Ingredients

4 (6 ounce) boneless beef sirloin steaks, room temperature
2 tablespoons olive oil
4 teaspoons cracked black pepper
2 teaspoons celery seed
1 1/2 cups extra spicy Bloody Mary mix
1 tablespoon orange juice concentrate
2 fluid ounces vodka
16 pitted green olives
3 tablespoons cold unsalted butter
2 teaspoons chopped garlic

Directions

Preheat a grill to medium heat.

Brush steaks on both sides with olive oil, then sprinkle with a mix of cracked pepper and celery seed. Cook steaks to desired doneness on the preheated grill. When done, allow steaks to rest on a plate while continuing with the recipe.

Bring the Bloody Mary mix, orange juice concentrate, and vodka to a boil over high heat; then reduce heat to medium, and simmer for 5 minutes. While sauce is cooking, puree the olives, butter, and garlic in a small food processor until almost smooth.

To serve, pour a pool of the sauce in the center of each plate. Slice each steak into 4 or 5 slices, and fan out over the sauce. Add a dollop of olive butter, and spoon a little more sauce overtop.

Lavender Pork Steaks

Ingredients

1 cup vegetable oil
4 tablespoons finely chopped fresh lavender
3 tablespoons chopped fresh rosemary
1 tablespoon chopped fresh thyme
4 pork steaks

Directions

Preheat an outdoor grill for low heat.

Pour oil into a large, resealable plastic bag. Add lavender, rosemary, and thyme; let stand for 10 minutes. Place steaks in bag with marinade, and marinate for 5 minutes.

Lightly oil grate. Remove steaks from marinade, and arrange on grill. Cook, turning once or twice, for 20 to 30 minutes, or until done.

Red Wine Reduction Steak Sauce

Ingredients

3 tablespoons butter
1/2 yellow onion, chopped
1/2 red onion, chopped
2 large shallots, chopped
2 tablespoons minced garlic
1 roma (plum) tomato, chopped
1 pound carrots, chopped
3/4 pound fresh mushrooms, sliced
1 (14 ounce) can beef broth
1 1/4 cups Merlot wine, divided

Directions

Heat the butter in a saucepan over medium-high heat; cook and stir the yellow and red onion, shallots, garlic, tomato, carrots, and mushrooms until the onions are translucent and the carrots have softened, 10 to 15 minutes. Pour in the beef broth and 1 cup of Merlot, and bring to a boil, scraping and dissolving any browned bits of flavor from the bottom of the pan. Reduce heat, and simmer until the vegetables are very soft and the pan juices have reduced by half, about 20 minutes.

Strain out and discard the vegetables from the sauce. Return the sauce to a boil over medium-high heat, stir in 1/4 cup of Merlot wine, and reduce heat. Simmer the sauce until it is reduced to 1/4 of its original volume, stirring occasionally, about 20 minutes.

Spinach Steak Pinwheels

Ingredients

1 1/2 pounds beef boneless sirloin steak
8 bacon strips, cooked and drained
1 (10 ounce) package frozen chopped spinach, thawed and squeezed dry
1/4 cup grated Parmesan cheese
1/2 teaspoon salt
1/8 teaspoon cayenne pepper

Directions

Make diagonal cuts in steak at 1-in. intervals to within 1/2 in. of bottom of meat. Repeat cuts in opposite direction. Pound to 1/2 in. thickness. Place bacon down the center of the meat. In a bowl, combine the spinach, Parmesan cheese, salt and cayenne; spoon over bacon. Roll up and secure with toothpicks. Cut into six slices.

Grill, uncovered, over medium heat for 6 minutes on each side or until meat reaches desired doneness (for medium-rare, a meat thermometer should read 145 degrees F; medium, 160 degrees F; well-done, 170 degrees F). Discard toothpicks.

Marinated Flank Steak

Ingredients

1/4 cup soy sauce
2 tablespoons vegetable oil
2 tablespoons tomato paste
1 garlic clove, minced
3/4 teaspoon dried oregano
3/4 teaspoon pepper
1 pound beef flank steak

Directions

In a large resealable plastic bag, combine the first six ingredients. Cut an 1/8-in.-deep diamond pattern into both sides of steak. Place in the bag; seal and turn to coat. Refrigerate overnight.

Drain and discard marinade. Place steak on a broiler pan. Broil 4 in. from the heat for 7-8 minutes on each side or until meat reaches desired doneness (for medium-rare, a meat thermometer should read 145 degrees F; medium, 160 degrees F; well-done, 170 degrees F).

Perfect Flat Iron Steak

Ingredients

2 pounds flat iron steak
2 1/2 tablespoons olive oil
2 cloves garlic, minced
1 teaspoon chopped fresh parsley
1/4 teaspoon chopped fresh rosemary
1/2 teaspoon chopped fresh chives
1/4 cup Cabernet Sauvignon
1/2 teaspoon salt
3/4 teaspoon ground black pepper
1/4 teaspoon dry mustard powder

Directions

Place the steak inside of a large resealable bag. In a small bowl, stir together the olive oil, garlic, parsley, rosemary, chives, Cabernet, salt, pepper and mustard powder. Pour over the steak in the bag. Press out as much air as you can and seal the bag. Marinate in the refrigerator for 2 to 3 hours.

Heat a nonstick skillet over medium-high heat. Fry the steak in the hot skillet for 3 to 4 minutes on each side, or to your desired degree of doneness. Discard the marinade. These steaks taste best at medium rare. Allow them to rest for about 5 minutes before serving.

Steak 'N' Onion Pie

Ingredients

2 tablespoons all-purpose flour
1 teaspoon salt
1/2 teaspoon pepper
1/2 teaspoon paprika
1/2 pound boneless beef top round steak, cut into 1/2 inch cubes
1 small onion, sliced and separated into rings
2 tablespoons vegetable oil
1 1/2 cups beef broth
1 cup cubed cooked potatoes
CRUST:
1 cup all-purpose flour
1/4 teaspoon salt
3 tablespoons cold butter or margarine
3 tablespoons shortening
2 tablespoons cold water
1 teaspoon milk

Directions

In a large resealable plastic bag, combine the flour, salt, pepper and paprika; mix well. Add beef, a few pieces at a time, and shake to coat.

In a skillet, cook beef and onion in oil until beef is browned and onion is tender. Add broth to the skillet. Bring to a boil. Reduce heat; cover and simmer for 45 minutes. Uncover; stir in the potatoes. Cook until heated through. Spoon meat mixture into a greased 7-in. pie plate or 2-cup baking dish.

For the crust, in a bowl, combine the flour and salt; cut in the butter and shortening until crumbly. Gradually add water, tossing with a fork until dough forms a ball. Roll out pastry to fit baking dish. Use a small cookie cutter to cut a shape in the center of the pastry; place pastry over meat mixture. Trim pastry to 1/2 in. beyond edge of dish; flute edges. Brush with milk. Bake at 375 degrees F for 35-40 minutes or until pastry is lightly browned on edges.

Cumin Lamb Steaks with Smashed Potatoes,

Ingredients

20 new potatoes, halved
1 tablespoon butter
2 cloves garlic, minced
2 tablespoons brown sugar
1 cup red wine

4 (6 ounce) lamb shoulder steaks
salt and pepper to taste
1 tablespoon cumin seeds
1 tablespoon vegetable oil

2 bunches fresh spinach, cleaned
1/4 cup sour cream
2 tablespoons softened butter

Directions

Place potatoes into a large saucepan and cover with salted water. Bring to a boil, then reduce heat to medium-low, cover, and simmer until tender, about 15 minutes. Drain and allow to steam dry for a minute or two.

Melt the butter in a saucepan over medium heat. Stir in the garlic, and cook for 3 to 4 minutes until the aroma of the garlic has mellowed. Add the brown sugar and red wine, then bring to a boil over medium-high heat. Allow to boil for 5 minutes, then remove from the heat, cover, and keep warm.

Meanwhile, season the lamb steaks with salt and pepper to taste. Press the cumin seeds into the steaks on both sides. Heat the vegetable oil in a large skillet over medium-high heat. Add the steaks, and cook on both sides until cooked to your desired degree of doneness, about 4 minutes per side for medium. Remove the steaks to rest in a warm spot. Place the spinach into the hot skillet, season to taste with salt and pepper, and cook until the spinach has wilted.

Mash the potatoes with the sour cream and butter; season to taste with salt and pepper. To serve, mound a serving of mashed potatoes onto the center of a dinner plate. Top with the spinach and a lamb steak. Strain the red wine sauce overtop.

Rock's T-Bone Steaks

Ingredients

4 teaspoons salt, or to taste
2 teaspoons paprika
1 1/2 teaspoons ground black pepper
3/4 teaspoon onion powder
3/4 teaspoon garlic powder, or to taste
3/4 teaspoon cayenne pepper, or to taste
3/4 teaspoon ground coriander, or to taste
3/4 teaspoon ground turmeric, or to taste
4 (16 ounce) t-bone steaks, at room temperature

Directions

Preheat an outdoor grill for high heat, and lightly oil the grate. Stir the salt, paprika, black pepper, onion powder, garlic powder, cayenne pepper, coriander, and turmeric together in a small bowl; set aside.

Rub the steaks on all sides with the seasoning mixture. Cook on the preheated grill to your desired degree of doneness, 3 to 3 1/2 minutes per side for medium-rare. An instant-read thermometer inserted into the center should read 130 degrees F (54 degrees C).

Firecracker Flank Steak

Ingredients

1 (16 ounce) jar Pace® Thick & Chunky Salsa
2 cups orange juice
1/2 cup olive oil
2 tablespoons packed brown sugar
2 tablespoons soy sauce
2 tablespoons Dijon-style mustard
1 teaspoon ground ginger root
2 pounds beef flank steak
Hot cooked rice
Chopped fresh parsley

Directions

Mix the salsa, orange juice, oil, sugar, soy, mustard and ginger in a nonmetallic shallow dish or large resealable plastic bag. Add the steak and turn it to coat with marinade. Cover the dish or seal the plastic bag and refrigerate for at least 1 hour or up to 24 hours.

Lightly oil the grill rack and heat the grill to medium. Grill steak until desired doneness, basting it frequently with marinade.

Heat the remaining marinade in a small saucepan over medium-high heat to a boil. Reduce the heat to low and cook for 10 minutes.

Slice the steak across the grain at a 45-degree angle to the cutting surface. Serve with the rice and the sauce. Top with the parsley.

Special Salmon Steaks

Ingredients

2 (8 ounce) salmon steaks
2 tablespoons butter or margarine, melted
2 tablespoons lemon juice
1 green onion, sliced
1 tablespoon minced fresh parsley
1/4 teaspoon garlic salt
1/8 teaspoon lemon-pepper seasoning

Directions

Place salmon in a lightly greased 8-in. square baking dish. Top with butter and lemon juice. Combine onion, parsley, garlic salt and lemon pepper; sprinkle over salmon. Bake, uncovered, at 400 degrees F for 15-20 minutes or until fish flakes easily with a fork.

Baked Fake Steak with Gravy

Ingredients

3 pounds ground beef
17 saltine crackers, finely crushed
1/2 cup milk
1 1/2 teaspoons garlic powder
1 1/2 teaspoons onion powder
1/4 teaspoon ground black pepper
1 pinch salt, or to taste
1/2 cup all-purpose flour
1 tablespoon vegetable oil
1 1/2 cups water
1 (10.75 ounce) can condensed beef and mushroom soup
1 (.75 ounce) packet dry brown gravy mix

Directions

In a large bowl, mix together the ground beef, saltine crackers and milk. Season with garlic powder, onion powder, salt and pepper, and mix until well blended. Line a 10x15 inch jellyroll pan with waxed paper. Press the beef mixture firmly into the pan. Cover with plastic wrap, and refrigerate 8 to 10 hours, or overnight.

Preheat the oven to 350 degrees F (175 degrees C). Remove plastic wrap from meat, and rub flour over the top side of the beef. Flip out of the pan onto waxed paper, and rub flour on the other side as well. Cut into pieces (I use a pizza cutter).

Heat oil in a large heavy skillet over medium-high heat. Fry the meat until browned on each side, turning only once. Remove to a 9x13 inch baking dish. In a medium bowl, mix together the water, condensed soup, and gravy mix. Pour over the meat in the dish. Cover the dish loosely with aluminum foil.

Bake for 1 hour in the preheated oven. Serve fake steak and gravy with potatoes, rice, or noodles.

Marinade for Steak I

Ingredients

1 cup vegetable oil
1/2 cup soy sauce
1/3 cup red wine vinegar
1/4 cup fresh lemon juice
3 tablespoons Worcestershire sauce
1 tablespoon freshly ground black pepper
2 tablespoons Dijon-style prepared mustard
1 onion, sliced
2 cloves garlic, minced

Directions

In a medium bowl, combine the oil, soy sauce, vinegar, lemon juice, Worcestershire sauce, ground black pepper, mustard, onion, and garlic. Mix together well, and use to marinate your favorite meat.

Sicilian Style Steak

Ingredients

- 1 cup Italian seasoned dry bread crumbs
- 1 cup grated Parmesan cheese
- 1 teaspoon seasoned salt
- 1 tablespoon garlic powder
- 1/2 cup olive oil
- 2 (16 ounce) t-bone steaks

Directions

Preheat an oven to 350 degrees F (175 degrees C). Lightly grease a broiler pan.

Stir the bread crumbs, Parmesan cheese, seasoned salt, and garlic powder together in a shallow dish such as a pie plate. Pour the olive oil into a separate shallow dish. Dip the t-bone steaks in the olive oil on both sides; allow excess to drip off. Press the steaks into the bread crumb mixture, and place onto the prepared broiler pan.

Bake on the middle rack in the preheated oven until the steaks have cooked to your desired degree of doneness, about 15 minutes for medium. An instant-read thermometer inserted into the center should read 140 degrees F (60 degrees C) for medium.

Chicken Fried Steak II

Ingredients

1 (5 ounce) can evaporated milk
2 1/2 tablespoons hot pepper sauce
3/4 teaspoon salt
2 cups all-purpose flour
2 1/2 teaspoons paprika 1/2 teaspoon garlic powder salt to taste
3/4 teaspoon ground black pepper
3 pounds round steak, pounded to about 1/2 inch thickness
4 cups vegetable oil

Directions

Combine the milk, hot pepper sauce and salt in a medium bowl. Measure one cup of flour into a second medium bowl. In a third medium bowl, combine the remaining flour, paprika, garlic powder, salt and ground black pepper.

First coat the steak in the unseasoned flour, then dip in the milk mixture, and finally coat meat in the seasoned flour. Repeat as necessary if there's more than one piece of meat.

Heat the oil in a medium skillet over medium high heat. Fry the coated meat in the oil for 3 minutes per side, or until golden brown. Drain meat on paper towels. (Note: Make sure the oil is fully heated before deep frying.)

Coffee Marinated Steak

Ingredients

2 tablespoons sesame seeds
3 tablespoons butter or margarine
1 medium onion, chopped
4 garlic cloves, minced
1 cup strong brewed coffee
1 cup soy sauce
2 tablespoons white vinegar
2 tablespoons Worcestershire sauce
2 pounds boneless beef top sirloin steak, cut 1 inch thick

Directions

In a skillet, toast sesame seeds in butter. Add onion and garlic; saute until tender. In a bowl, combine the coffee, soy sauce, vinegar, Worcestershire sauce and sesame seed mixture. Pour half into a large resealable plastic bag; add steak. Seal bag and turn to coat; refrigerate for 8 hours or overnight, turning occasionally. Cover and refrigerate remaining marinade.

Drain and discard marinade from steak. Grill steak, covered, over medium-hot heat for 6-10 minutes on each side or until meat reaches desired doneness (for medium-rare, a meat thermometer should read 145 degrees F; medium, 160 degrees F; well-done, 170 degrees F). Warm reserved marinade and serve with steak.

Smoky Steak Marinade

Ingredients

- 1/2 cup Worcestershire sauce
- 1/4 cup liquid smoke
- 1 1/2 tablespoons salt
- 3 tablespoons seasoned salt
- 2 tablespoons garlic powder
- 2 1/2 tablespoons onion powder

Directions

Whisk together Worcestershire sauce, liquid smoke, salt, seasoned salt, garlic powder, and onion powder in a bowl until the salts have dissolved.

To use, pour the marinade over up to 2 pounds of meat in a resealable plastic bag. Seal the bag, and refrigerate overnight. The following morning, discard the marinade, and cook the meat as desired.

Rosemary Steak

Ingredients

1 cup red wine
1 teaspoon salt
1 sprig fresh rosemary
4 New York strip steaks, cut 1-inch thick

Directions

Combine the red wine, salt and rosemary in a small bowl. Let stand at room temperature for 2 to 3 hours.

Heat a large griddle or cast-iron skillet over high heat. Place the steaks on the hot pan, and cook for about 8 minutes per side, or to desired degree of doneness. The internal temperature should be at least 145 degrees F (62 degrees C) for medium rare. Pour in the wine mixture, and allow it to boil for a minute. Serve steaks with sauce on a deep platter.

Seasoned Flank Steak

Ingredients

1/4 cup vegetable oil
2 tablespoons water
1 tablespoon lemon-pepper seasoning
1 teaspoon seasoned salt
1 (1 1/2-pound) beef flank steak

Directions

In a large resealable plastic bag, combine the first four ingredients; add steak. Seal bag and turn to coat; refrigerate for 1-2 hours, turning occasionally.

Grill steak, uncovered, over medium-hot heat for 6-12 minutes or until meat reaches desired doneness (for medium-rare, a meat thermometer should read 145 degrees F; medium, 160 degrees F; well-done, 170 degrees F).

Doreen's Steak Marinade

Ingredients

- 1/3 cup sherry
- 1/3 cup soy sauce
- 1/3 cup vegetable oil
- 2 tablespoons honey
- 2 tablespoons grated fresh ginger root
- 1 clove garlic, minced

Directions

In a medium bowl, mix sherry, soy sauce, vegetable oil, honey, ginger, and garlic. Marinate steaks for at least 4 hours before grilling as desired.

Spinach-Stuffed Steak

Ingredients

1 (10 ounce) package frozen chopped spinach, thawed and drained
1 (7 ounce) jar roasted red peppers, drained
1 egg white
1/2 cup seasoned bread crumbs
1/4 cup grated Parmesan cheese
1/4 cup sunflower kernels, toasted
1 garlic clove, minced
1/2 teaspoon salt
1 (1 1/2-pound) flank steak

Directions

In a bowl, combine the first eight ingredients; mix well.

Cut steak horizontally from a long edge to within 1/2 in. of opposite edge; open (like a book) and flatten to 1/2-in. thickness. Spread spinach mixture over the steak to within 1 in. of edges. Roll up, jelly-roll style, starting with a long side; tie with kitchen string. Place in a greased 13-in. x 9-in. x 2-in. baking dish.

Cover and bake at 350 degrees for 1 hour. Uncover; bake 30-45 minutes longer or until tender. Let stand for 10-15 minutes. Cut into 1/2-in. slices.

Mock Chicken Fried Steak

Ingredients

- 1 pound ground beef
- 2 teaspoons chopped fresh parsley
- 1 tablespoon chili powder
- 1 teaspoon salt
- 1 egg
- 2 cups crushed saltine crackers, divided
- 1/2 cup oil for frying

Directions

In a medium bowl, mix together the ground beef, parsley, chili powder, salt, egg, and 1 cup of crushed saltine crackers. Form into 6 balls, then flatten into patties. Coat patties with remaining cracker crumbs, and place them on a plate. Refrigerate for at least 30 minutes.

Heat the oil in a large skillet over medium heat. Fry patties for about 7 minutes per side, or until the centers are well done and the outside is golden brown.

Marinated Sirloin Steak

Ingredients

1 cup lemon-lime soda
3/4 cup vegetable oil
3/4 cup soy sauce
1/4 cup lemon juice
1 teaspoon garlic powder
1 teaspoon prepared horseradish
1 pound boneless beef sirloin steak

Directions

In a large resealable plastic bag, combine the first six ingredients. Add steak and turn to coat. Seal and refrigerate 8 hours or overnight, turning occasionally.

Drain and discard marinade. Grill steaks, covered, over medium-hot heat for 3-5 minutes on each side or until meat reaches desired doneness (for medium-rare, a meat thermometer should read 145 degrees F; medium, 160 degrees F; well-done, 170 degrees F).

Creole Pan-Fried Flat Iron Steak

Ingredients

2 pounds flat iron steak
1 tablespoon hot pepper sauce (e.g. Tabascoв„ў)
2 tablespoons lime juice
2 teaspoons garlic salt
1/8 teaspoon salt
1/8 teaspoon ground black pepper
2 1/4 teaspoons blackened seasoning
1/2 cup butter
1/2 cup water

Directions

Heat a skillet over medium heat. Season the steak with hot pepper sauce. Sprinkle or mist with a little lime juice and season lightly with just a portion of the garlic salt, salt, black pepper and blackened seasoning.

Place the steak in the pan and cover with a lid. Cook for about 20 minutes, or to your desired degree of doneness, turning and adding more seasoning every 5 minutes.

Remove steaks to a serving platter and keep warm. Stir butter and water into the pan, removing any browned bits from the bottom to make a gravy. Season with additional garlic salt, salt and pepper to taste. Serve steaks with gravy drizzled over them.

Lemon Basil Pesto Flat Iron Steak

Ingredients

4 cloves garlic
2 cups packed fresh basil leaves
1/3 cup pine nuts
1/2 cup extra-virgin olive oil
1/2 cup freshly grated Parmesan cheese
1 1/2 tablespoons fresh lemon juice
3/4 teaspoon red pepper flakes
6 (6 ounce) flat iron steaks
2 large cloves garlic, minced
salt and pepper to taste

Directions

Chop 4 garlic cloves in a food processor until minced. Add the basil and pine nuts, and pulse a few times to combine. With the food processor running, slowly pour in the olive oil, stopping once or twice to scrape down the sides. Place the Parmesan cheese, lemon juice, and red pepper flakes into the food processor, and pulse until blended. Season to taste with salt and pepper.

Rub the flat iron steaks with 2 cloves minced garlic, season to taste with salt and pepper, then set aside. Preheat an outdoor grill for medium-high heat and lightly oil grate.

Grill the steaks to desired degree of doneness on preheated grill, about 4 minutes per side for medium. Baste the steaks occasionally with a little of the pesto sauce. Once done, serve topped with the remaining pesto.

Fiesta Grilled Ham Steak

Ingredients

- 1 (2 pound) Cook'sB® brand Bone-In Thick Cut Ham Steak
- 3/4 cup jalapeno pepper jelly
- 2 cloves garlic, minced
- 1/4 cup chopped cilantro

Directions

Preheat charcoal or gas grill. In a small saucepan, heat jelly and garlic over medium heat until jelly is melted (or, in a microwave-safe bowl, heat in microwave oven at high power until melted, about 1 minute). Stir in cilantro. Set aside 1/4 cup mixture for serving.

Place ham steaks on grill over medium heat. Grill 3 minutes. Turn ham steaks; brush with half of remaining jelly mixture and continue to grill 3 minutes. Turn again; brush with remaining half of jelly mixture and continue to grill 1 to 2 minutes or until ham is glazed and heated through. Serve with reserved jelly mixture.

Pepper Steak and Rice

Ingredients

1 cup uncooked long-grain white rice
2 cups water
2 tablespoons olive oil
1 medium onion, sliced and separated into rings
1/2 green bell pepper, julienned
1 pound boneless sirloin steak, cut into thin strips
2 cloves garlic, peeled and chopped
1 teaspoon browning sauce
1 tablespoon ground paprika
seasoning salt to taste
ground black pepper to taste
1 1/2 cups water
2 tablespoons cornstarch
1/2 cup water

Directions

Place rice and 2 cups water in a medium saucepan, and bring to a boil. Cover, reduce heat, and simmer 20 minutes.

Heat olive oil in a medium saucepan over medium heat, and saute onion and green bell pepper until tender.

Stir steak, garlic, and browning sauce into the onion and green bell pepper mixture. Season with paprika, seasoning salt, and black pepper. Cook and stir until steak is evenly browned. Mix in 1 1/2 cups water, and bring to a boil.

In a small bowl, dissolve cornstarch in 1/2 cup water. Stir into the boiling steak mixture until thickened. Serve over the cooked rice.

Tasty Tuna Steak

Ingredients

1 tablespoon olive oil
1 1/2 teaspoons whole fennel seeds
3 cloves garlic, minced
1 red bell pepper, cut into thin strips
3/4 cube fish bouillon, crushed
1/2 lemon, juiced
2 tablespoons dry white wine
1 head baby bok choy, cleaned and sliced

salt and black pepper to taste
1 1/2 teaspoons fennel seeds, crushed
1 (8 ounce) tuna steak
1 tablespoon olive oil

Directions

Heat 1 tablespoon of olive oil in a skillet over medium heat. Stir in 1 1/2 teaspoons of whole fennel seeds, and cook until they bubble and begin to pop, about 30 seconds. Stir in the garlic and red bell pepper; cook and stir for 2 minutes. Stir in the fish bouillon until dissolved, then add the lemon juice, white wine, and bok choy. Cook and stir until the bok choy is tender, about 5 minutes.

Meanwhile, combine some salt and pepper with the crushed fennel seeds on a plate. Press the tuna steak into the salt mixture on both sides. Heat the remaining tablespoon of olive oil in a separate skillet over high heat. Place the tuna steak in the skillet, and cook until browned on both sides and cooked to your desired degree of doneness, about 45 seconds per side for rare.

Cut the tuna into 1/4-inch thick slices and arrange onto a serving platter. Top with the bok choy mixture to serve.

John's Mango Steak

Ingredients

1/4 cup olive oil
1/4 cup minced apple
1/2 cup diced honeydew
1/2 cup diced mango
1 tablespoon garlic salt
2 tablespoons Worcestershire sauce
2 teaspoons kosher salt
1/4 teaspoon hot pepper sauce
1 tablespoon ground black pepper
6 pounds beef steaks

Directions

In a small saucepan over low heat, combine the oil, apple, honeydew, mango, garlic salt, Worcestershire sauce, kosher salt, hot pepper sauce to taste and ground black pepper.

Heat for about 5 minutes to get warm. Place the steak in a shallow nonporous dish. Cover with the marinade and refrigerate, covered, for at least 3 hours. Flip steak over halfway through marinating.

Preheat an outdoor grill for high heat and lightly oil grate.

Grill steak for 10 minutes per side, dousing with remaining marinade, if desired. Steak is done when internal temperature reaches at least 145 degrees F (63 degrees C).

Sesame Sirloin Steak

Ingredients

- 1/4 cup soy sauce
- 2 tablespoons sesame seeds, toasted
- 2 garlic cloves, minced
- 2 tablespoons olive or vegetable oil
- 2 tablespoons brown sugar
- 1/4 teaspoon pepper
- 1 dash hot pepper sauce
- 3/4 pound (3/4 inch thick) boneless beef sirloin steak

Directions

In a large resealable plastic bag, combine the soy sauce, sesame seeds, garlic, oil, brown sugar, pepper and hot pepper sauce. Pierce steak on both sides with a fork; place in the bag. Seal and turn to coat; refrigerate for 8 hours or overnight.

Drain and discard marinade. Grill the steak, covered, over medium heat for 7-9 minutes on each side or until meat reaches desired doneness (for medium-rare, a meat thermometer should read 145 degrees F; medium, 160 degrees F; well-done, 170 degrees F).

President Ford's Braised Eye Round Steak

Ingredients

2 tablespoons vegetable oil
2 large onions, sliced
12 (4 ounce) beef eye of round steaks
1/4 teaspoon dried thyme
1 teaspoon seasoned salt
1/4 cup all-purpose flour for coating
1 cup beef consomme
1 cup Burgundy wine
1 teaspoon chopped fresh parsley

Directions

Heat the oil in a large skillet over medium-high heat. Add onions; cook and stir until lightly browned and tender, about 5 minutes. Remove the onions from the skillet using a slotted spoon and set aside in a bowl. Season the steaks with thyme and seasoned salt, then dust them lightly with flour. Fry the steaks in the skillet over medium-high heat until browned on each side, about 5 minutes per side.

Pour the red wine and beef consomme in with the beef. Return the cooked onions to the pan. Cook over medium-high heat until the aroma of wine dissipates, 2 to 3 minutes. Reduce heat to low, cover, and simmer for 1 hour. Serve steaks with the sauce and a garnish of fresh parsley.

Slow-Cooked Flank Steak

Ingredients

1 (1 1/2-pound) flank steak, cut in half
1 tablespoon vegetable oil
1 large onion, sliced
1/3 cup water
1 (4 ounce) can chopped green chilies
2 tablespoons vinegar
1 1/4 teaspoons chili powder
1 teaspoon garlic powder
1/2 teaspoon sugar
1/2 teaspoon salt
1/8 teaspoon pepper

Directions

In a skillet, brown steak in oil; transfer to a slow cooker. In the same skillet, saute onion for 1 minute. Gradually add water, stirring to loosen browned bits from pan. Add remaining ingredients; bring to a boil. Pour over the flank steak. Cover and cook on low for 7-8 hours or until the meat is tender. Slice the meat; serve with onion and pan juices.

Kicky Steak Strips with Rice

Ingredients

1/2 cup Worcestershire sauce
2 tablespoons yellow mustard
1 pound top sirloin steak, cut into thin strips
1 cup uncooked long-grain white rice
2 cups water
1 tablespoon olive oil
1/2 cup chopped sweet onion
2 cloves garlic, peeled and chopped
1 teaspoon pepper

Directions

In a medium container, mix Worcestershire sauce and mustard. Place steak strips in the mixture. Cover, and marinate in the refrigerator at least 30 minutes.

Place rice and water in a medium saucepan, and bring to a boil. Reduce heat, cover, and cook 20 minutes.

Heat olive oil in a medium saucepan over medium heat. Stir in the onion and garlic, and cook until tender. Season with pepper. Place steak into the saucepan and cook 5 to 7 minutes on each side, to desired doneness. Discard remaining marinade. Serve over the cooked rice.

Steak Salad

Ingredients

- 1 3/4 pounds beef sirloin steak
- 1/3 cup olive oil
- 3 tablespoons red wine vinegar
- 2 tablespoons lemon juice
- 1 clove garlic, minced
- 1/2 teaspoon salt
- 1/8 teaspoon ground black pepper
- 1 teaspoon Worcestershire sauce
- 3/4 cup crumbled blue cheese
- 3 cups romaine lettuce - rinsed, dried, and torn into bite-size pieces
- 2 tomatoes, sliced
- 1 small green bell pepper, sliced
- 1 carrot, sliced
- 1/2 cup sliced red onion
- 1/4 cup sliced pimento-stuffed green olives

Directions

Preheat grill for high heat.

Lightly oil grate. Place steak on grill and cook for 3 to 5 minutes per side or until desired doneness is reached. Remove from heat and let sit until cool enough to handle. Slice steak into bite size pieces.

In a small bowl, whisk together the olive oil, vinegar, lemon juice, garlic, salt, pepper and Worcestershire sauce. Mix in the cheese. Cover and place dressing in refrigerator.

Onto chilled plates arrange the lettuce, tomato, pepper, onion and olives. Top with steak and drizzle with dressing. Serve with crusty grilled French bread. Enjoy!

Halibut Steaks

Ingredients

1 tablespoon olive oil
1 small onion, halved and thinly sliced
1/2 bell pepper, sliced thinly
8 ounces sliced fresh mushrooms
1 clove chopped fresh garlic
2 medium zucchini, julienned
6 (6 ounce) halibut steaks
1/2 teaspoon dried basil
1/2 teaspoon salt, or to taste
1/2 teaspoon ground black pepper
1 medium tomato, thinly sliced

Directions

Preheat the oven to 400 degrees F (200 degrees C).

Heat the olive oil in a skillet over medium heat. Add the onion, bell pepper, mushrooms, garlic and zucchini. Cover, and cook stirring occasionally, until the onions are translucent, about 5 minutes.

Place halibut steaks into a shallow baking dish, and top with the sauteed vegetables. Season with basil, salt and pepper.

Bake for 10 minutes in the preheated oven, then remove the dish, and cover the fillets with a layer of sliced tomato. Return to the oven, and bake for an additional 10 minutes, or until fish flakes easily with a fork.

Steaks With Roquefort Sauce

Ingredients

2 tablespoons butter
1 tablespoon olive oil
4 (5 ounce) beef sirloin steaks
salt and coarsely ground black pepper to taste
2 tablespoons brandy
1 cup heavy cream
3 ounces Roquefort cheese, crumbled
Italian flat leaf parsley, for garnish

Directions

Melt the butter and heat the oil in a skillet over high heat. Season steaks with salt and pepper, and quickly sear on both sides. Reduce heat to medium, and continue cooking steaks 5 minutes on each side, or to desired doneness. Remove from skillet and keep warm.

Pour brandy into the skillet and stir to loosen browned bits from bottom. Stir in cream, and return to a boil. Cook and stir until sauce is thick enough to coat the back of a spoon. Mix cheese into the sauce until melted. Pour over the steaks to serve. Garnish steaks with parsley.

Steakhouse Wheat Bread for the Bread Machine

Ingredients

3/4 cup warm water
1 tablespoon butter, softened
1/4 cup honey
1/2 teaspoon salt
1 teaspoon instant coffee granules
1 tablespoon unsweetened cocoa powder
1 tablespoon white sugar
1 cup bread flour
1 cup whole wheat flour
1 1/4 teaspoons bread machine yeast

Directions

Place the warm water, butter, honey, salt, coffee, cocoa, sugar, bread flour, whole wheat flour, and bread machine yeast in the pan of a bread machine in the order listed. Put on regular or basic cycle with light crust.

Cheddar Mushroom Pork Steaks

Ingredients

1 (10.75 ounce) can condensed cream of mushroom soup
1 (11 ounce) can condensed cheese soup
2 (10.75 ounce) cans milk
3 thick cut pork steaks
1 tablespoon dried oregano
1 tablespoon dried basil
salt and pepper to taste

Directions

Preheat oven to 375 degrees F (190 degrees C).

In a large bowl, combine the mushroom soup, Cheddar cheese soup and the milk. Mix until well blended. Season the pork steaks with the oregano, basil and salt and pepper to taste.

Pour about 2 cups of the sauce into a 9x13 inch baking dish and place the pork steaks over the sauce. Top the steaks with the remaining sauce.

Bake, uncovered, at 375 degrees F (190 degrees C) for 1 hour, then turn steaks over, making sure they're always covered with the sauce, and bake for another 30 minutes.

Steak on a Stick

Ingredients

1/2 cup soy sauce
1/4 cup olive oil
1/4 cup water
2 tablespoons molasses
2 teaspoons mustard powder
1 teaspoon ground ginger
1/2 teaspoon garlic powder
1/2 teaspoon onion powder
2 pounds flank steak, cut into thin strips
32 wooden skewers (8 inch long) soaked in water

Directions

In a large resealable bag, combine the soy sauce, olive oil, water, molasses, mustard powder, ginger, garlic powder and onion powder. Seal and shake the bag to mix together. Add steak strips to the bag and seal. Refrigerate for at least 8 hours to marinate.

Preheat the oven's broiler. Thread meat onto skewers and place on a broiling rack.

Broil the steak for 3 to 4 minutes on each side. Arrange on a platter to serve.

Comforting Cube Steaks

Ingredients

4 (4 ounce) cube steaks
1/2 teaspoon Cajun seasoning, or to taste
1/4 teaspoon freshly ground black pepper
1 (12 fluid ounce) can or bottle lemon-lime flavored carbonated beverage
2 (10.75 ounce) cans condensed cream of mushroom soup
1 (1 ounce) envelope dry onion soup mix

Directions

Preheat the oven to 325 degrees F (165 degrees C). Grease a 9x13 inch baking dish.

Season the steaks on both sides with Cajun seasoning and black pepper. Place the steaks into the prepared baking dish. Pour the lemon-lime beverage over them. Combine the cream of mushroom soup and dry onion soup mix, and pour over the steaks.

Bake, uncovered, for about 1 hour, or until meat reaches desired doneness. Do not open the oven door during the first hour of cooking. Serve steaks with gravy spooned over.

CPSIA information can be obtained
at www.ICGtesting.com
Printed in the USA
LVHW022326150621
690293LV00012B/748